"nature itself is the best physician"
- Hippocrates

For thousands of years, people have been using nature as folk remedies and to heal themselves. From aches and pains to serious illness, people have turned to the healing properties of the earth for guidance.

Today, we still harness the gifts that Mother Nature provides to heal our minds, bodies, and spirits. This holistic way of healing brings us back to our origins as a species, as we work with the forces of the natural world rather than against it.

Inspired by the most popular natural remedies, this coloring book connects you back to your roots of using nature as medicine.

Follow Holistic Sage on Facebook to stay up to date on new products.

Copyright © 2020 by Holistic Sage.
All rights reserved. No part of this book may be reproduced in any manner without written permission.

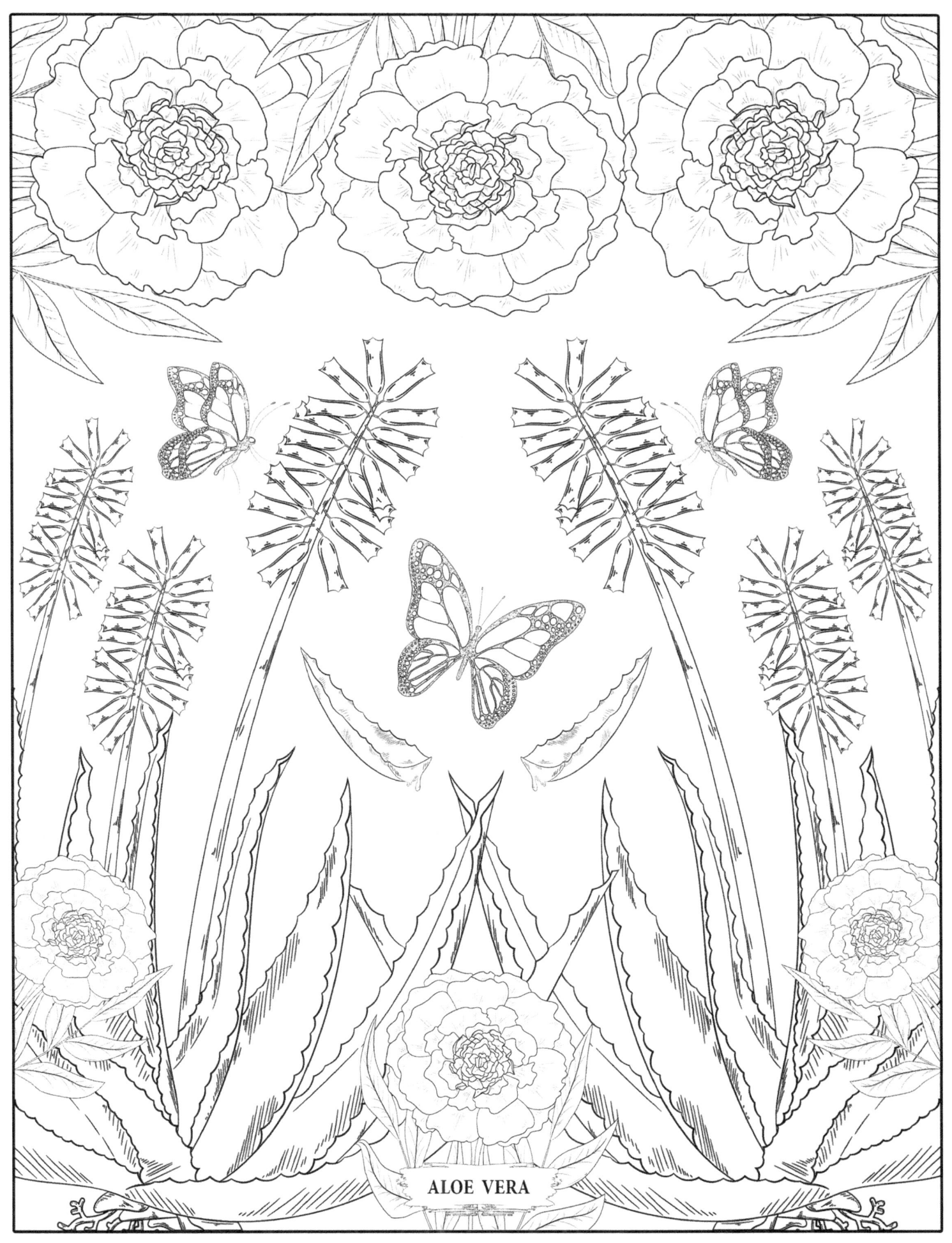
ALOE VERA

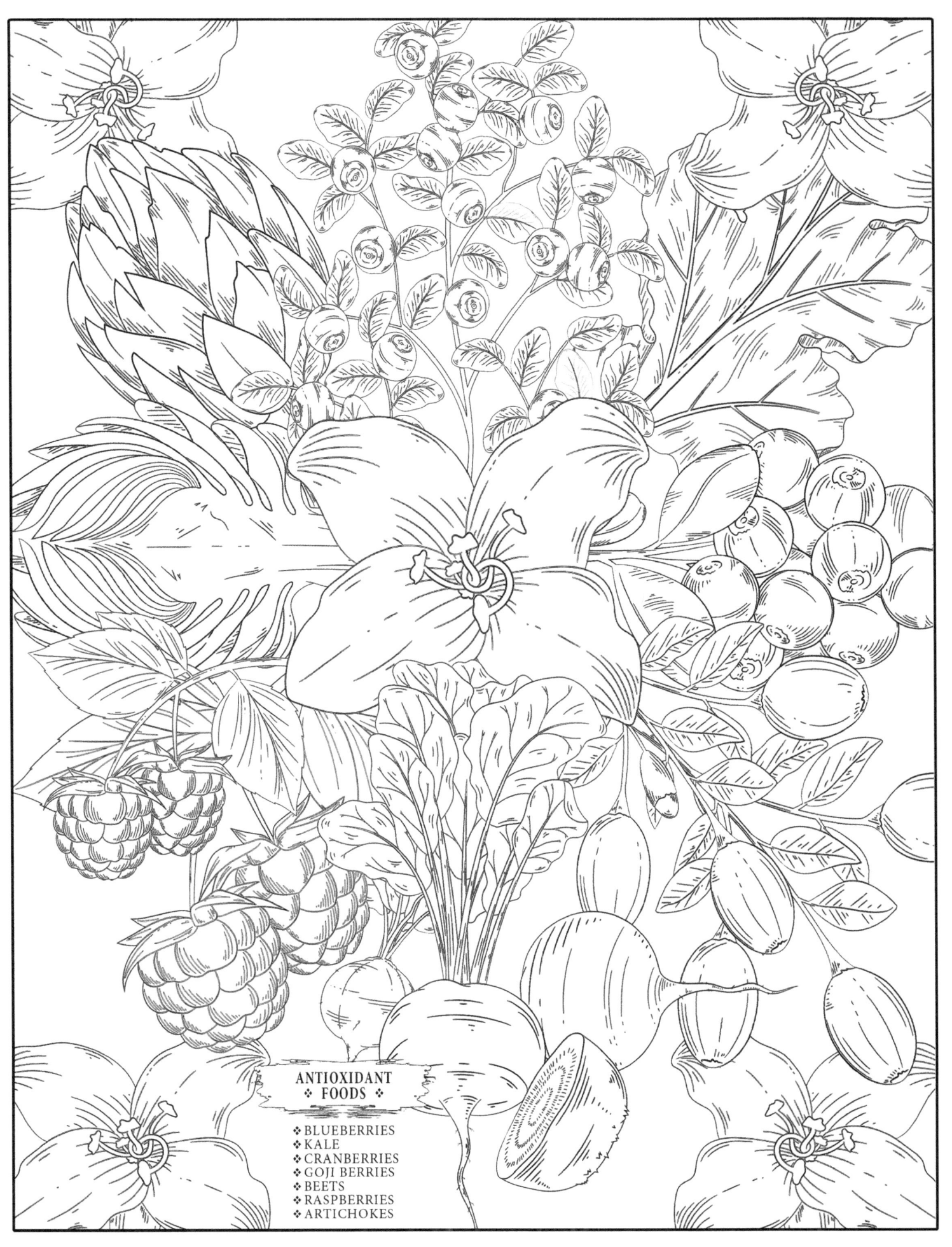

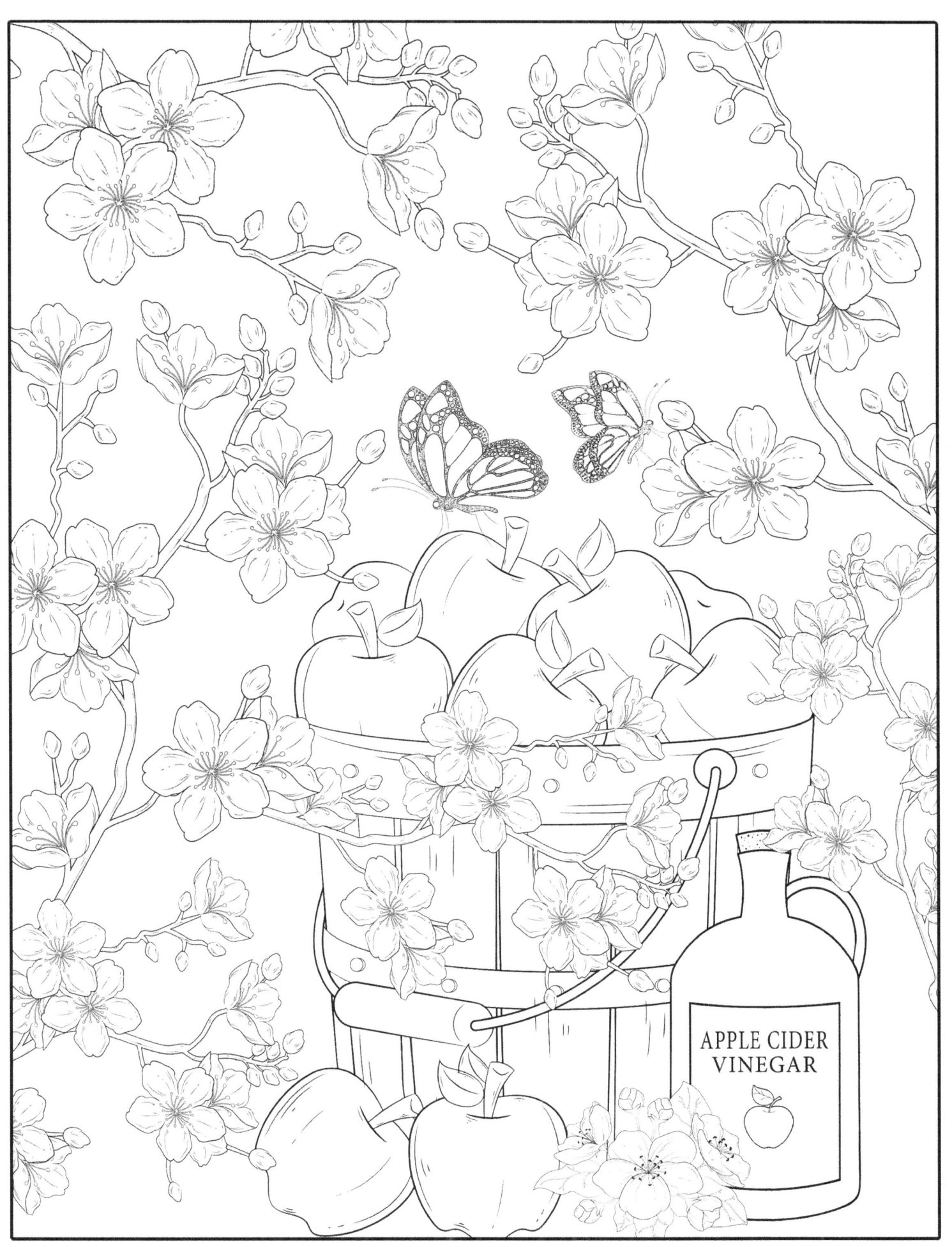

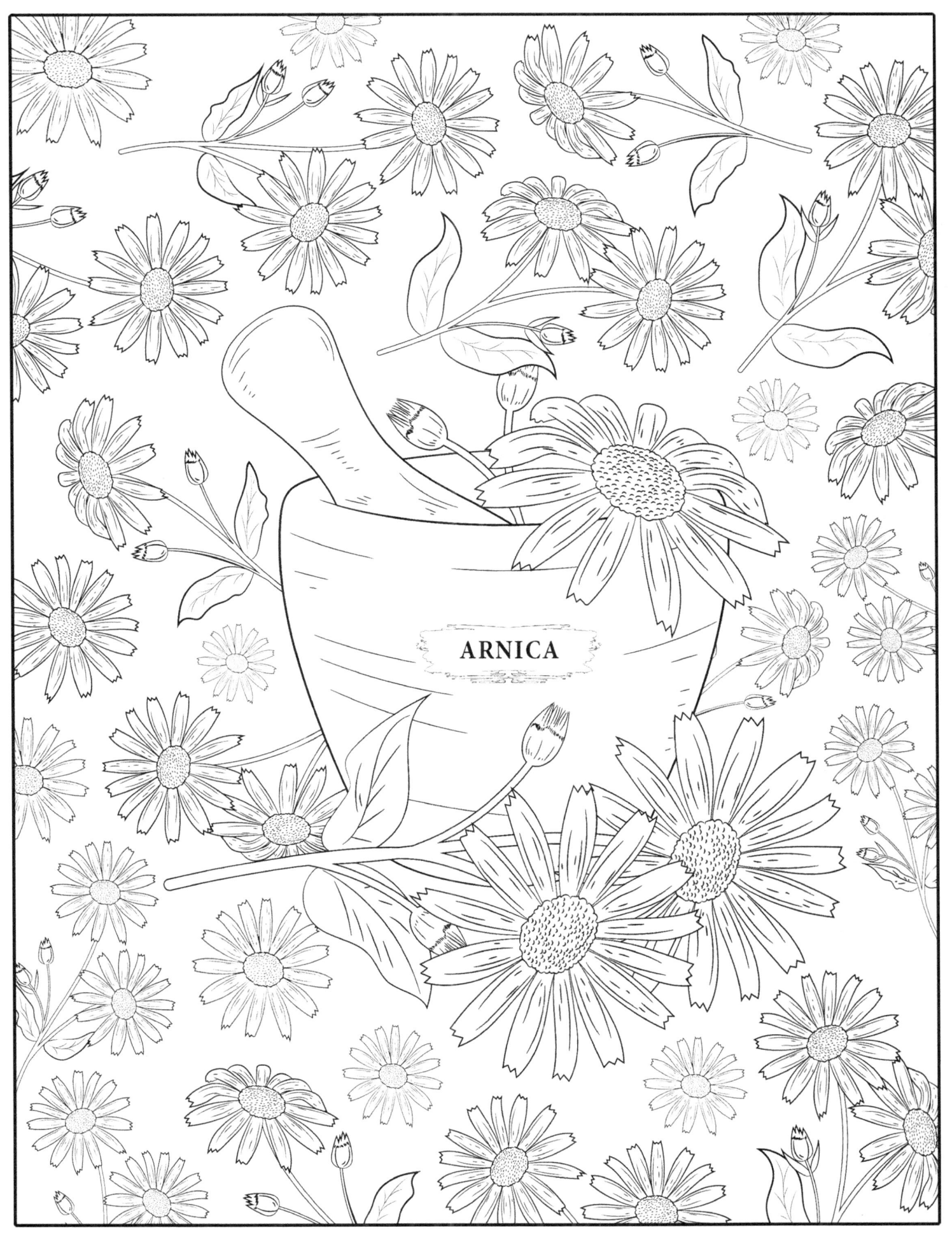

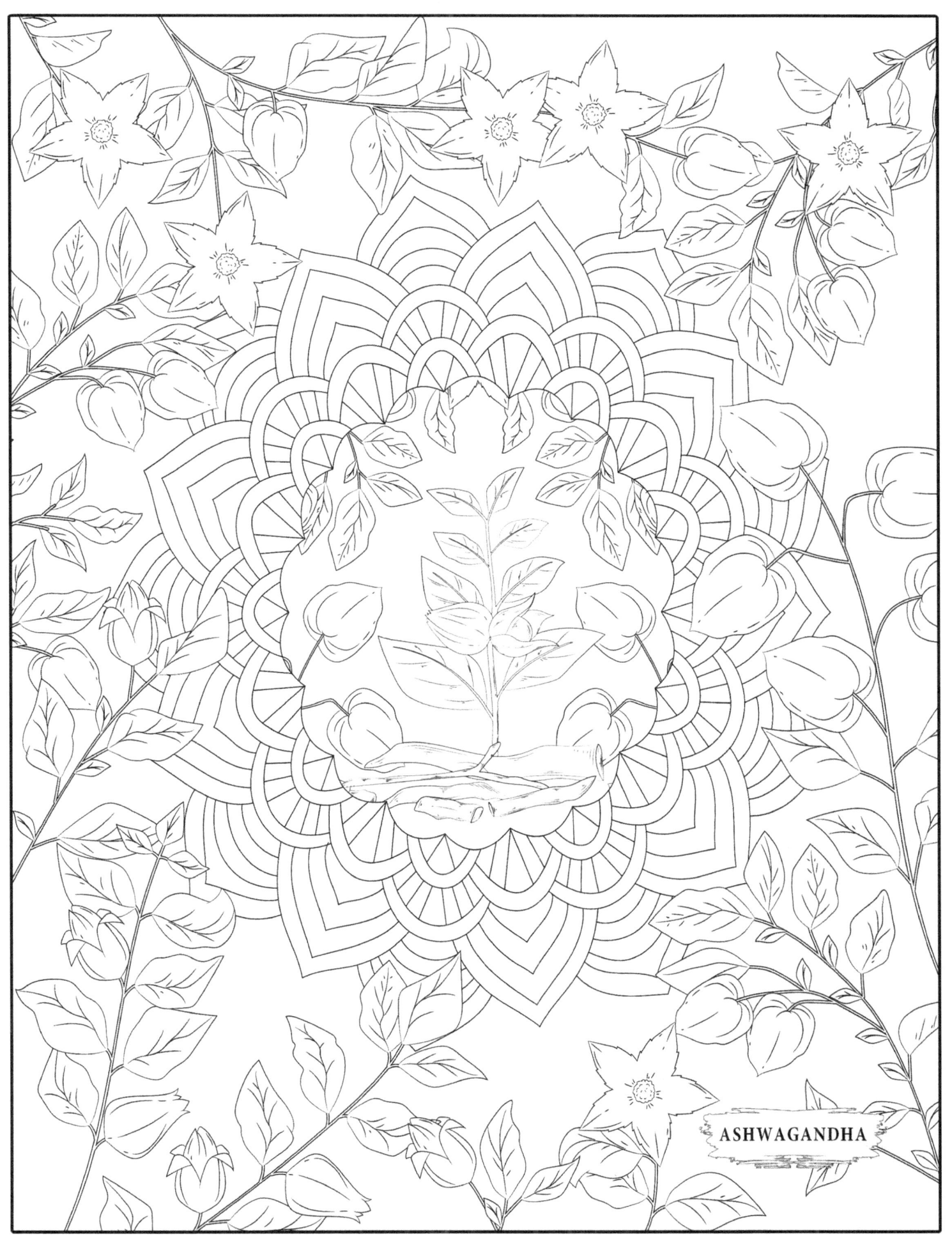

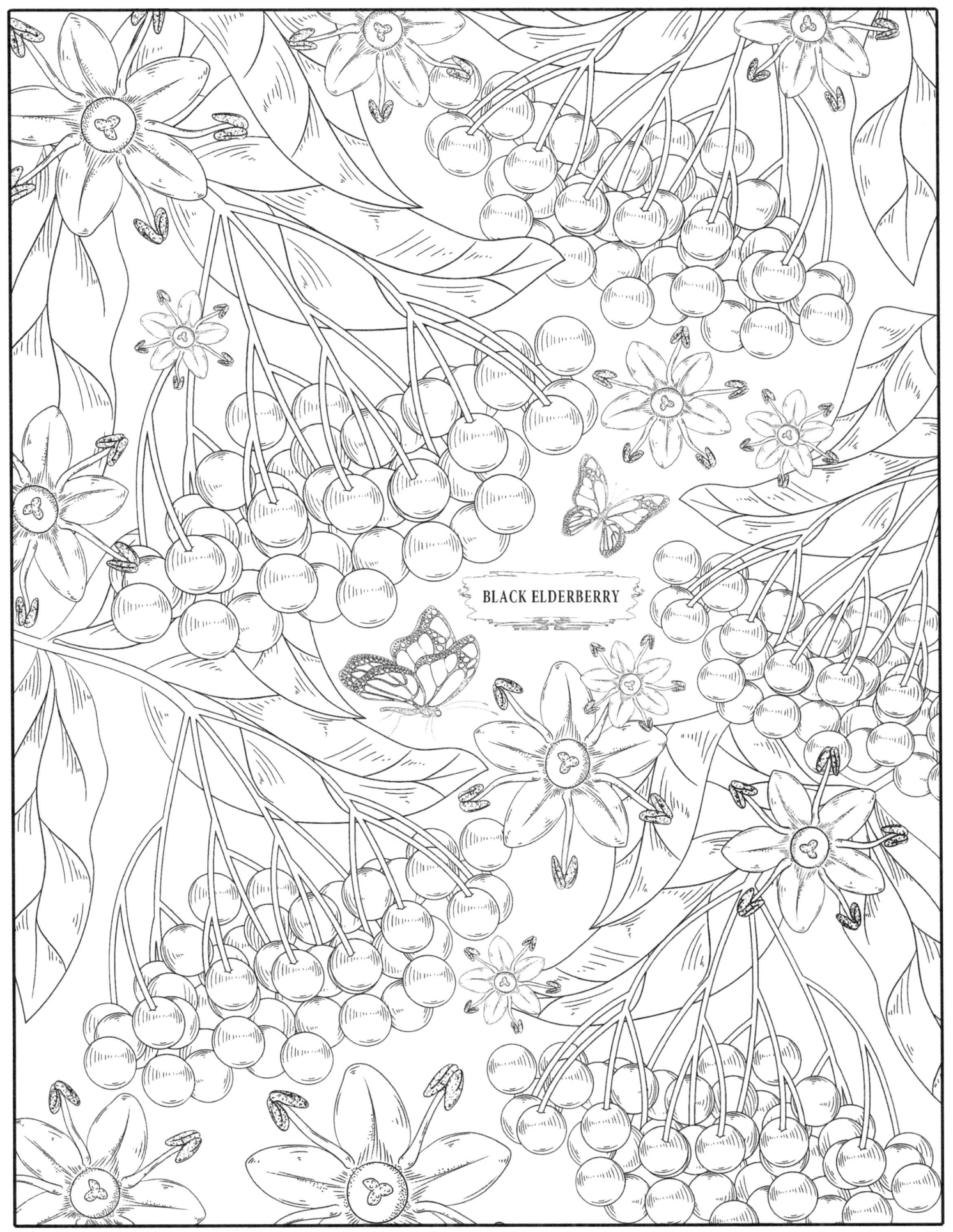

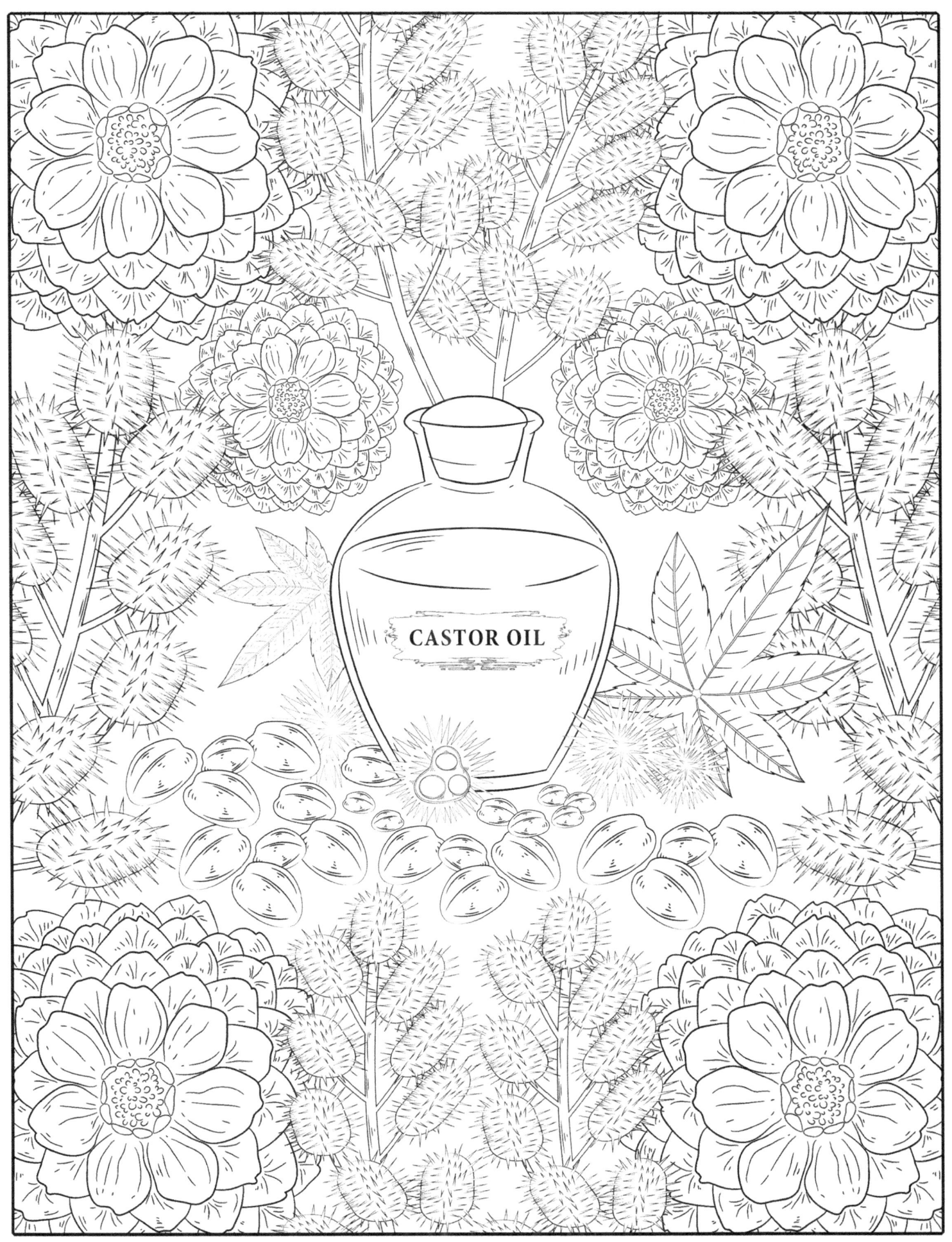

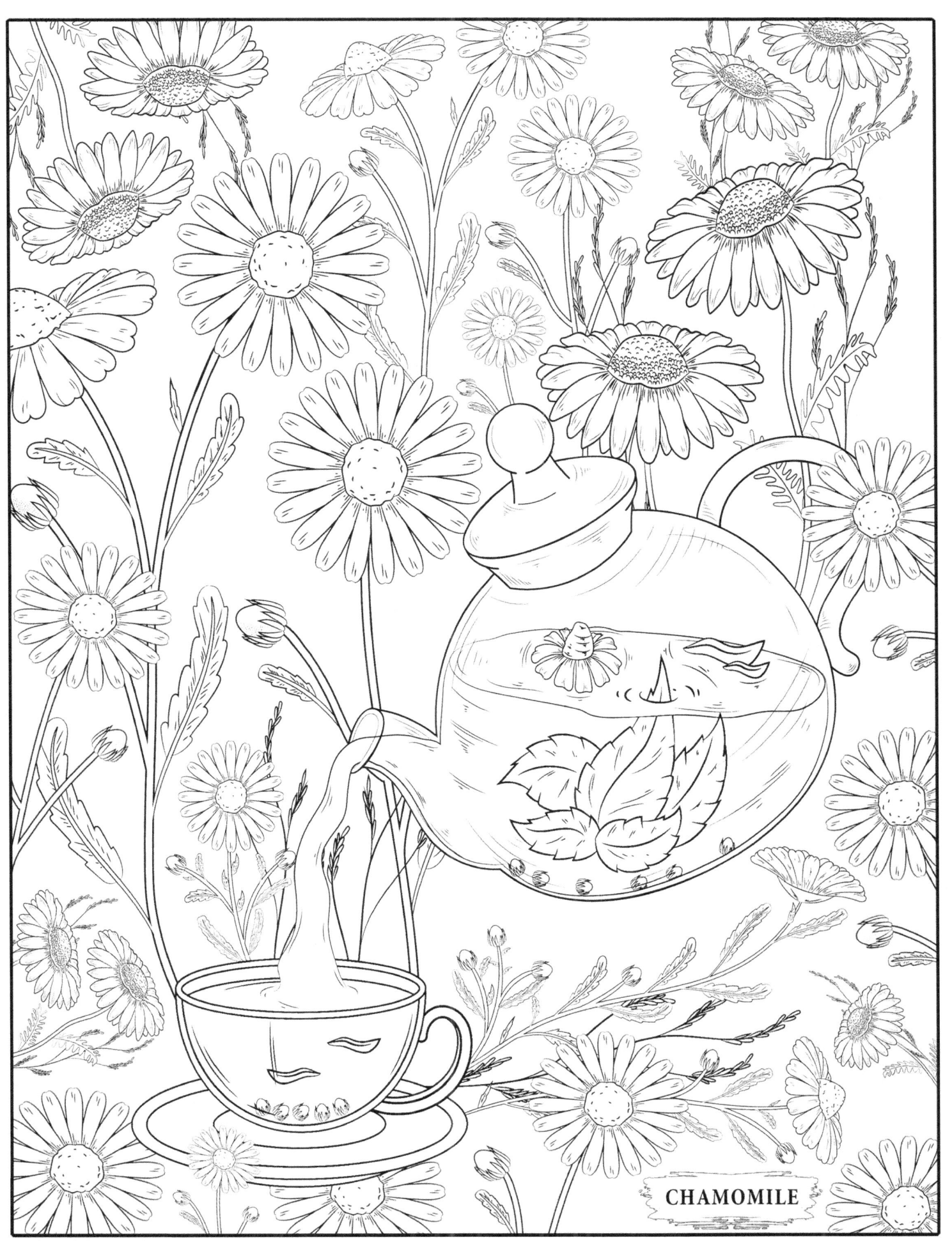

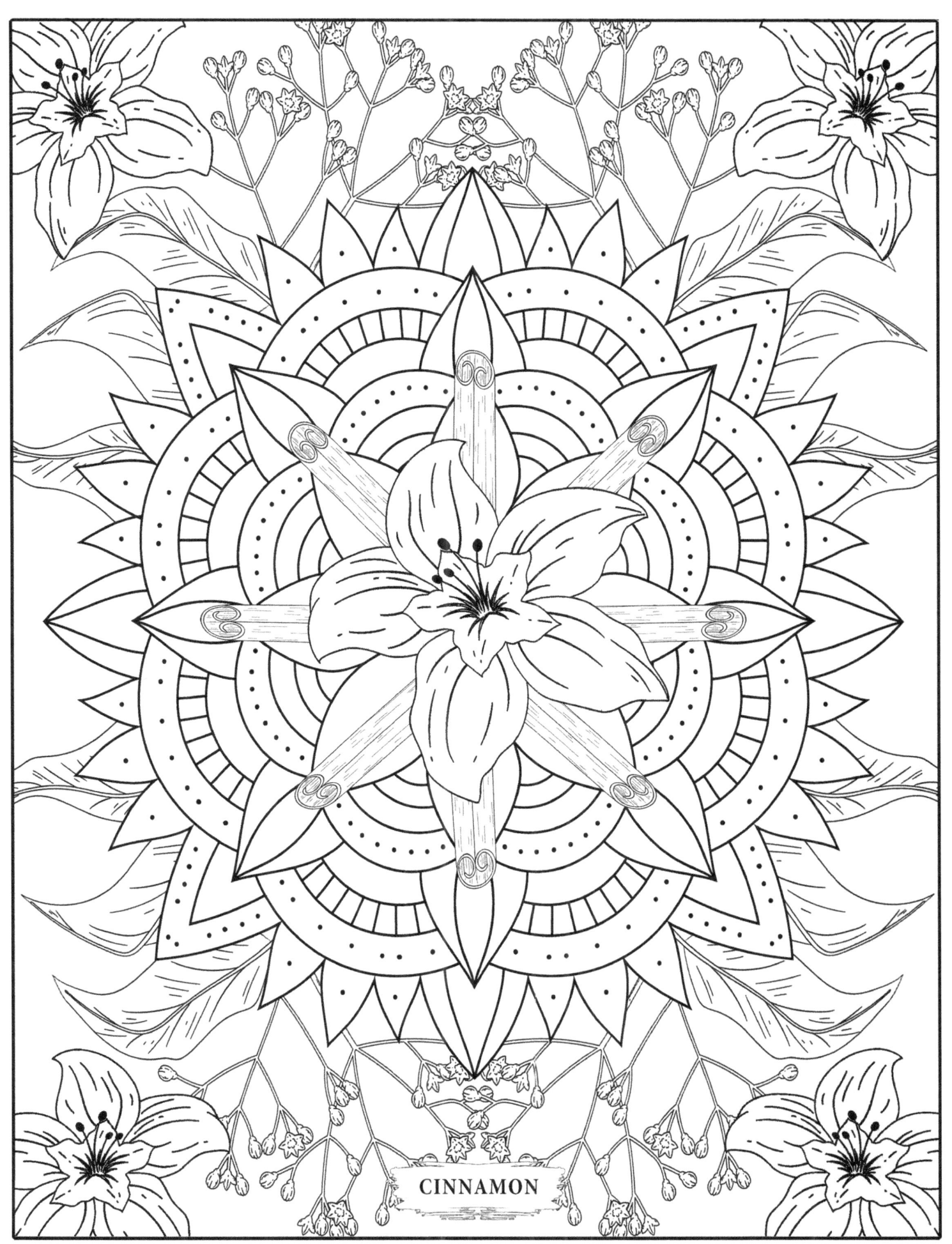

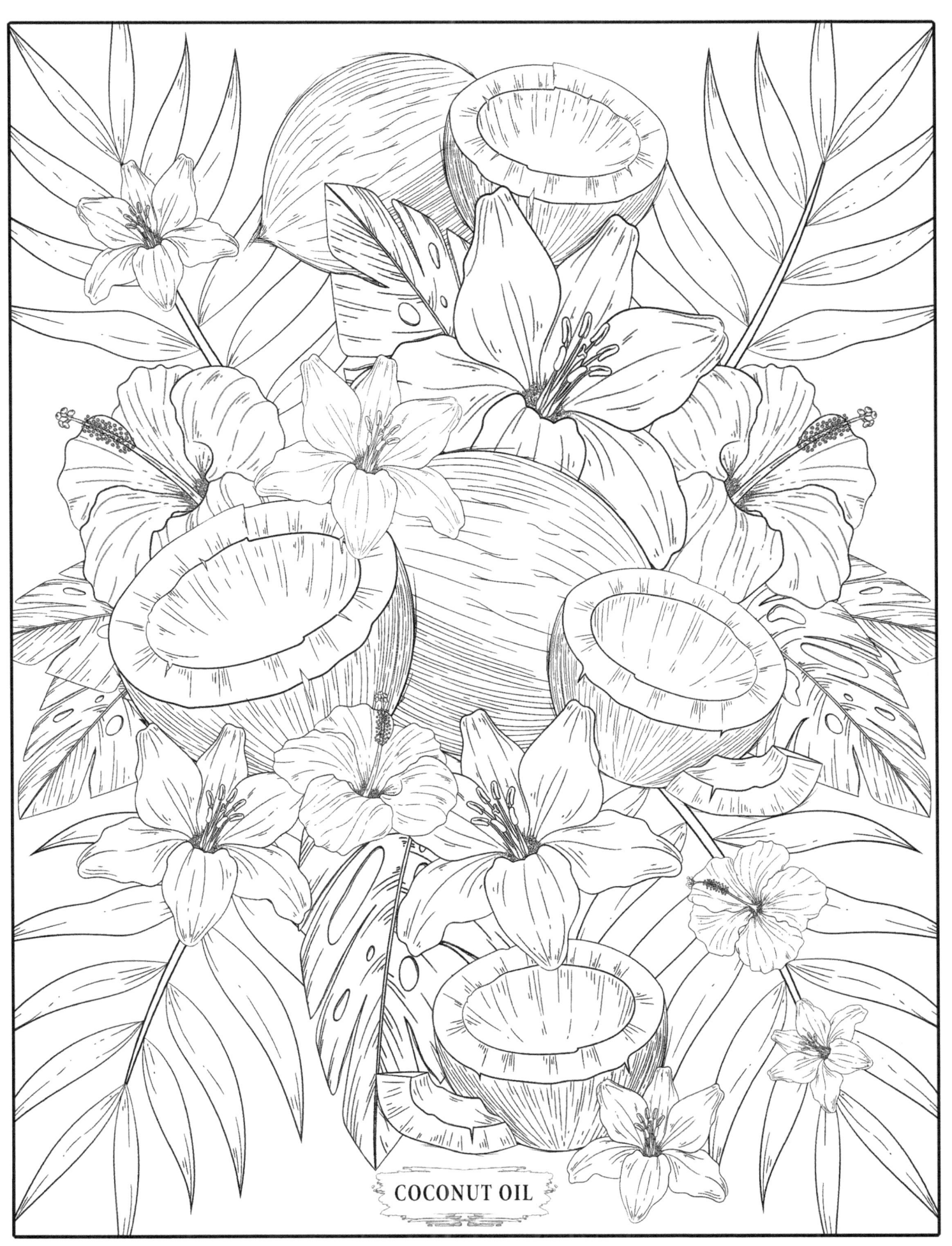

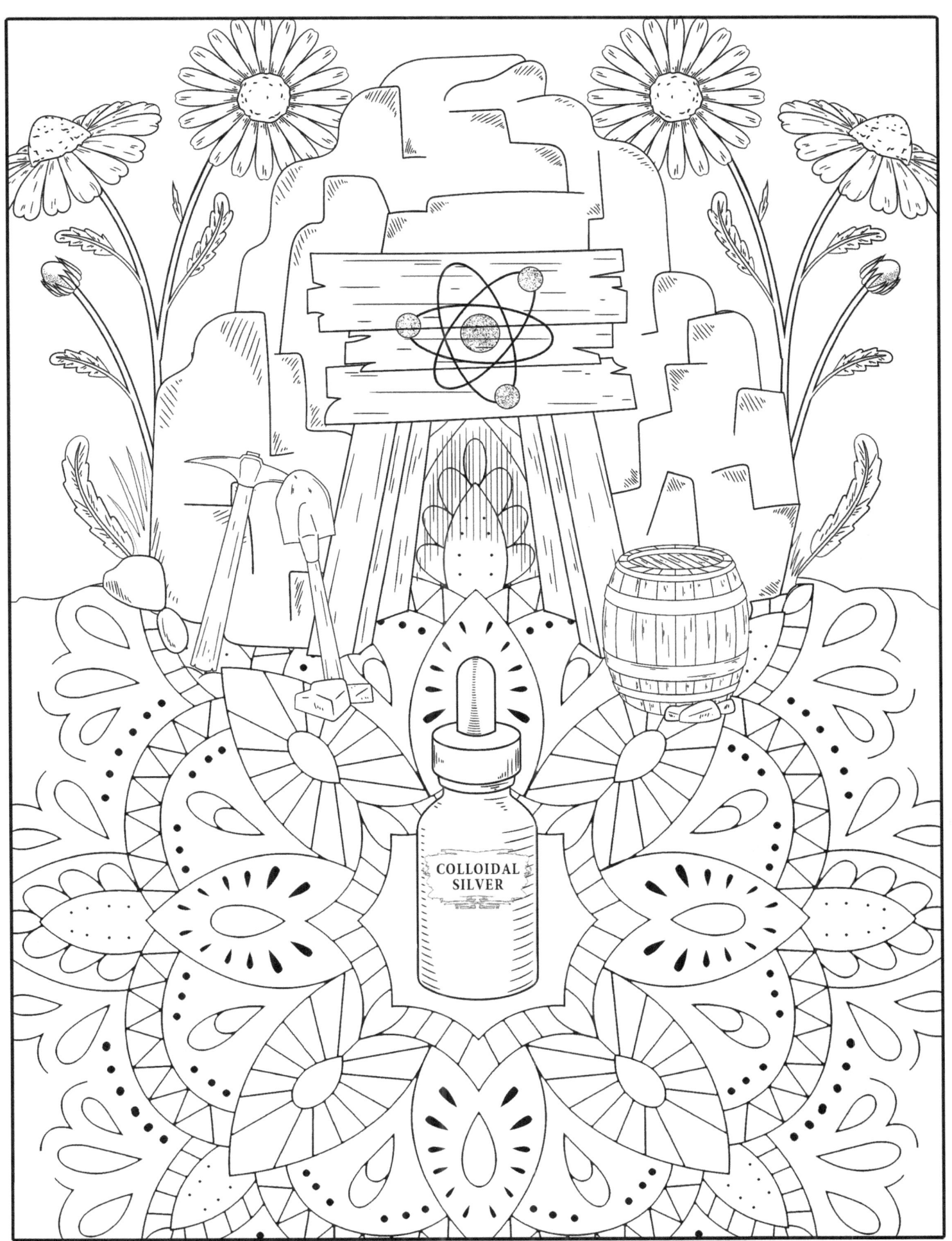

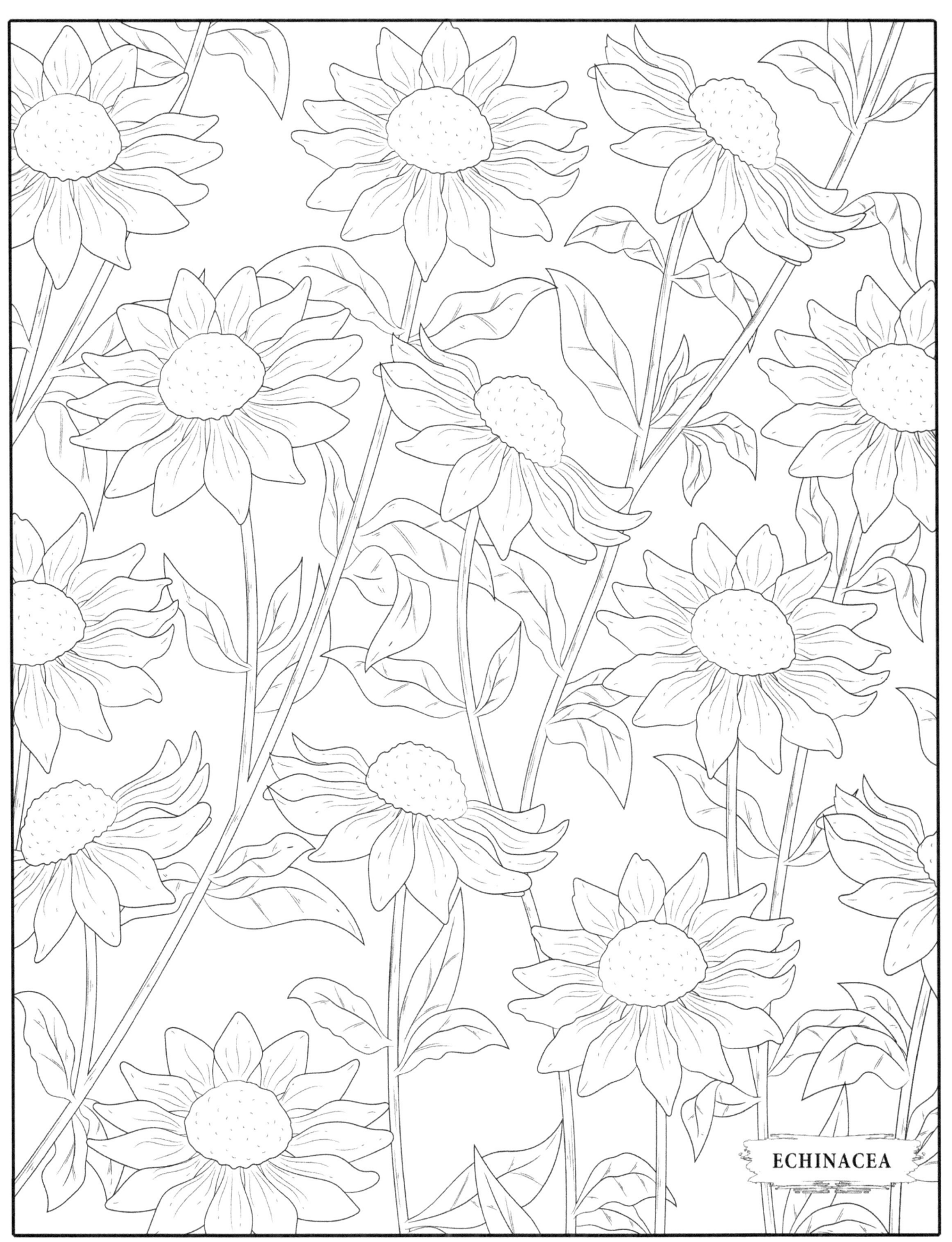

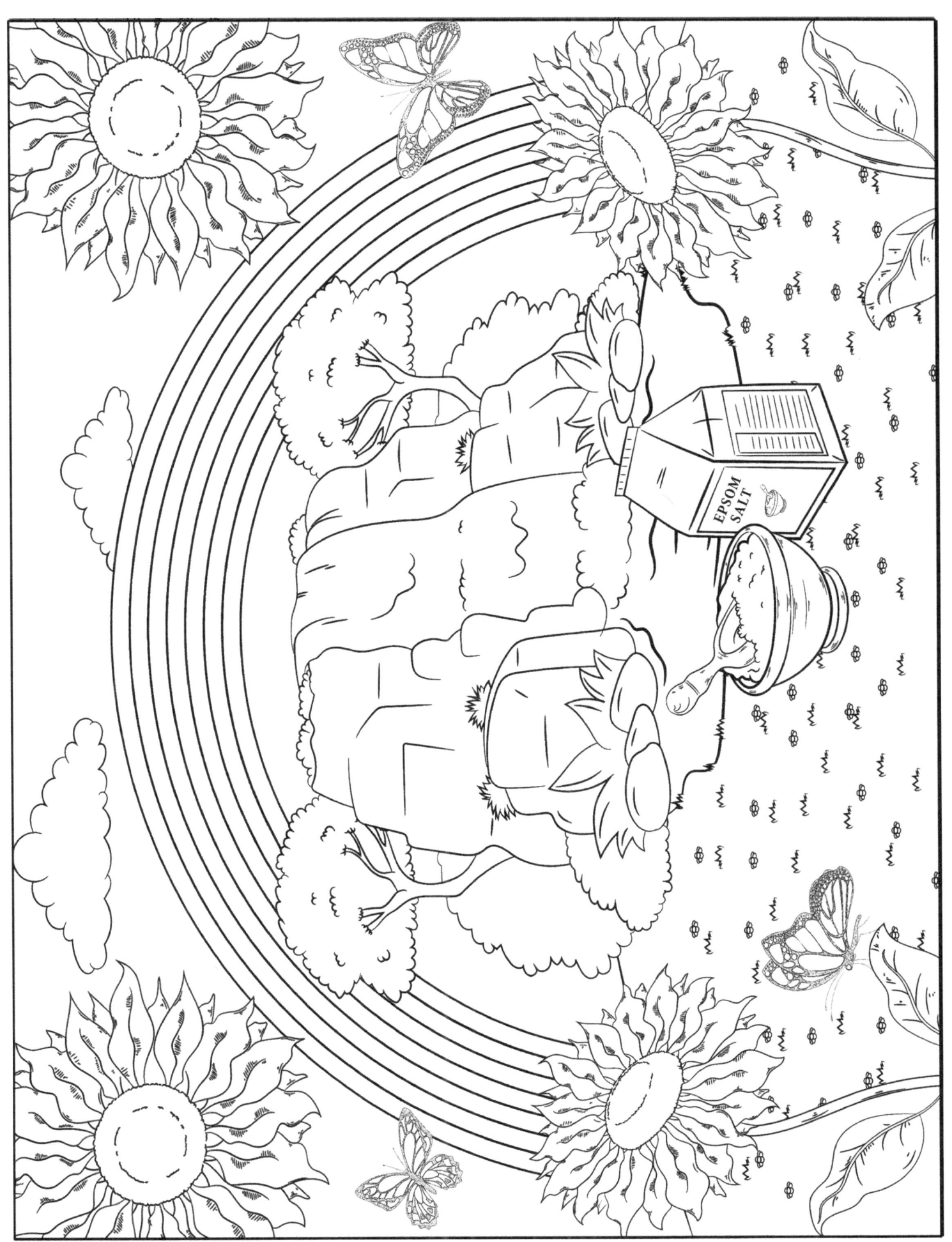

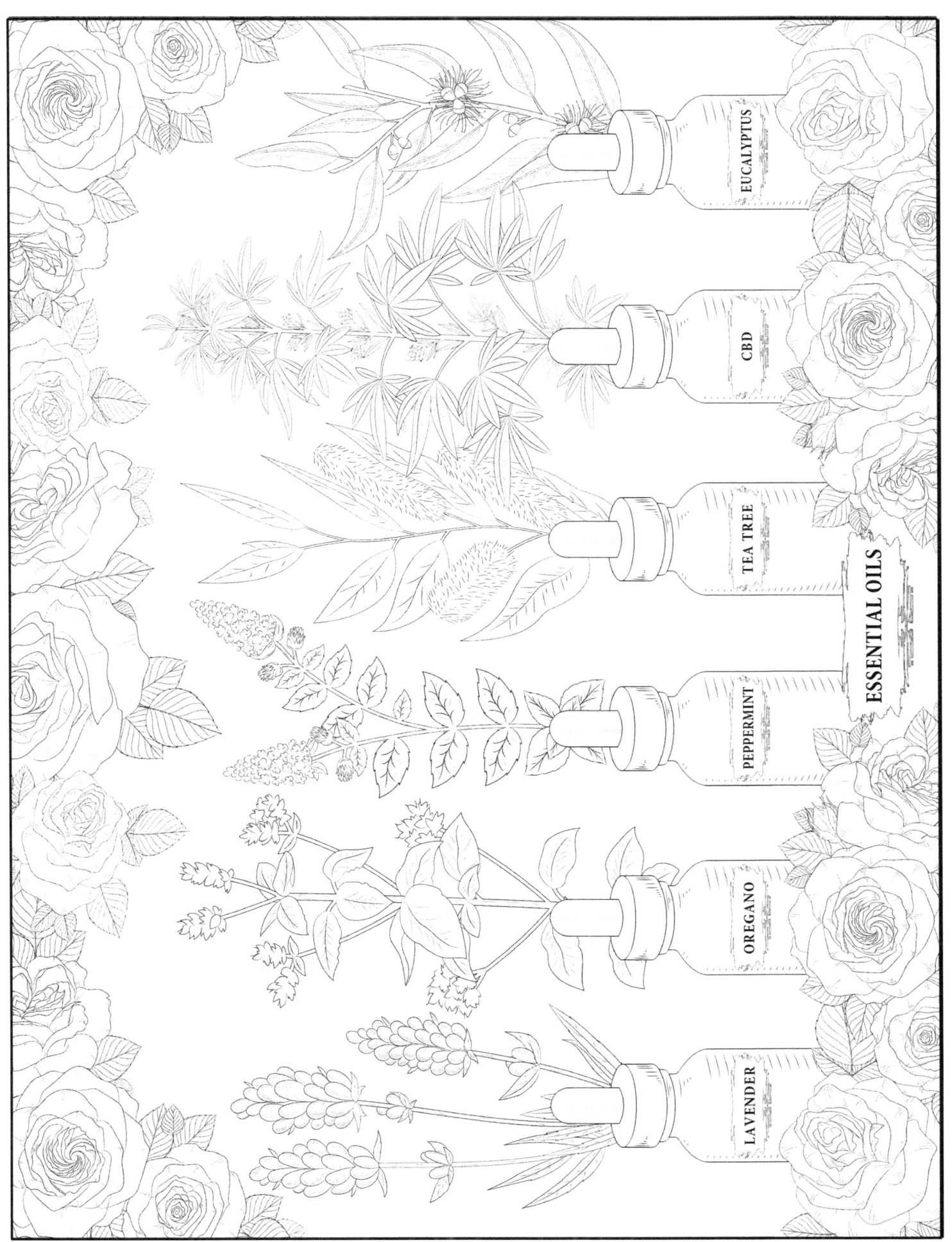

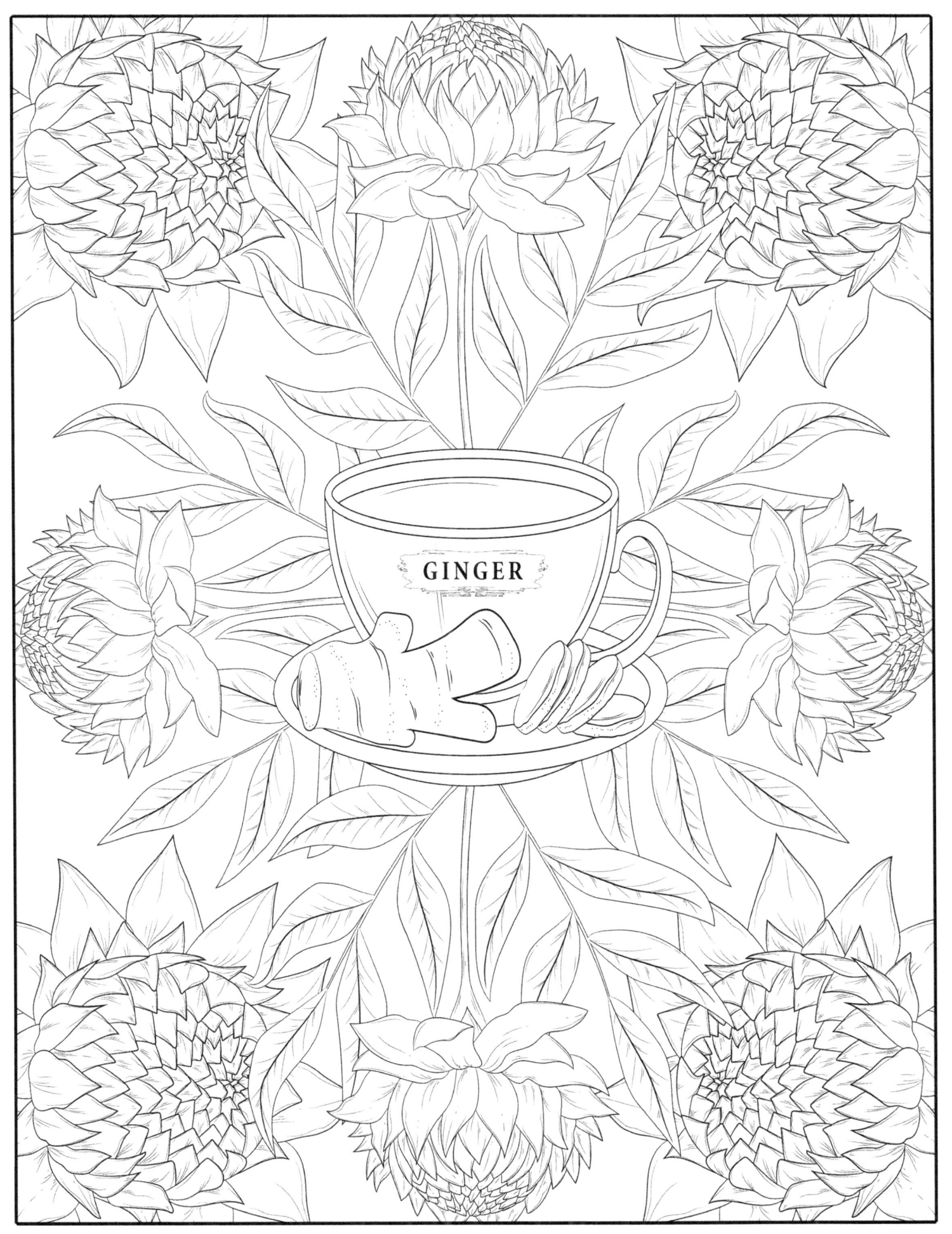

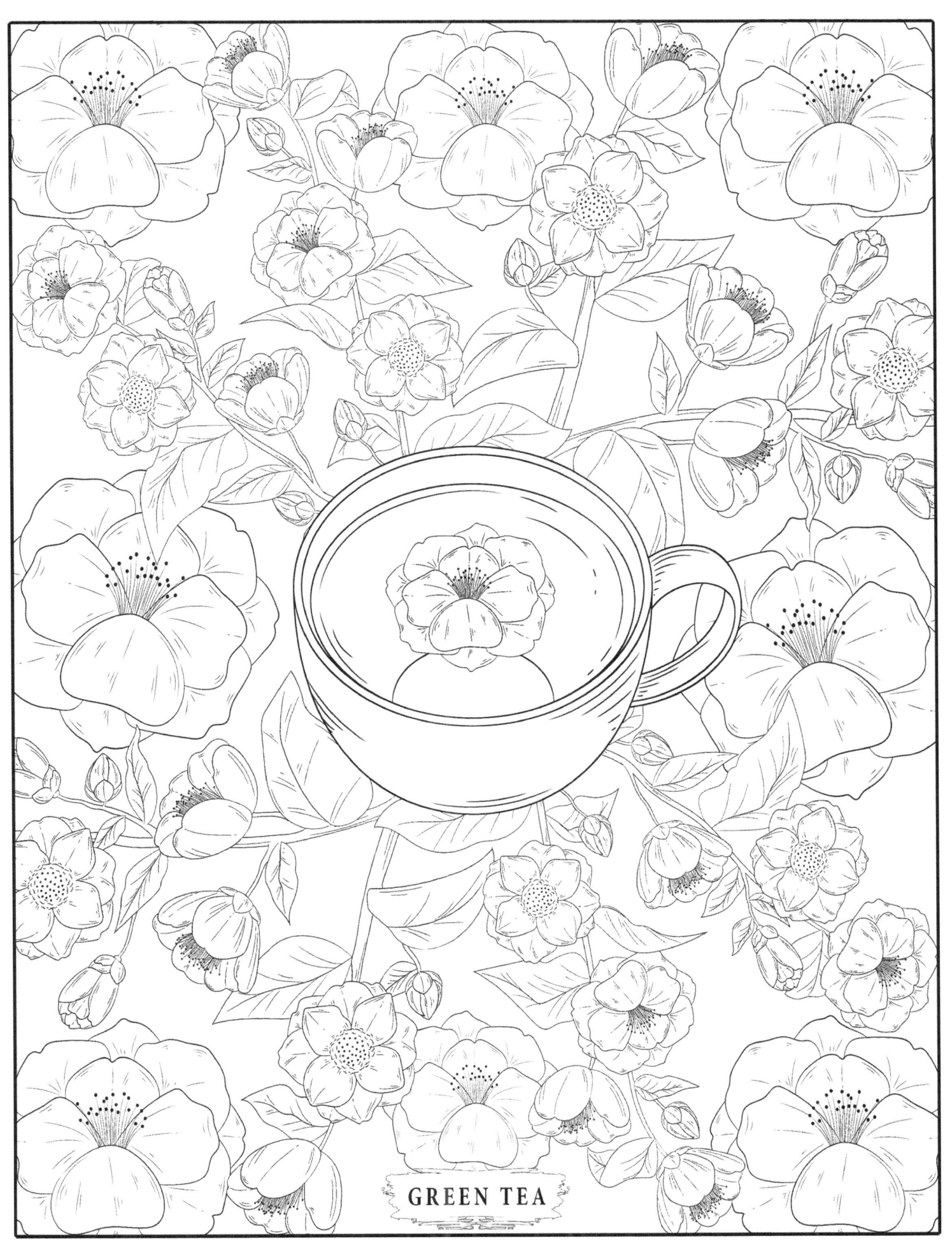

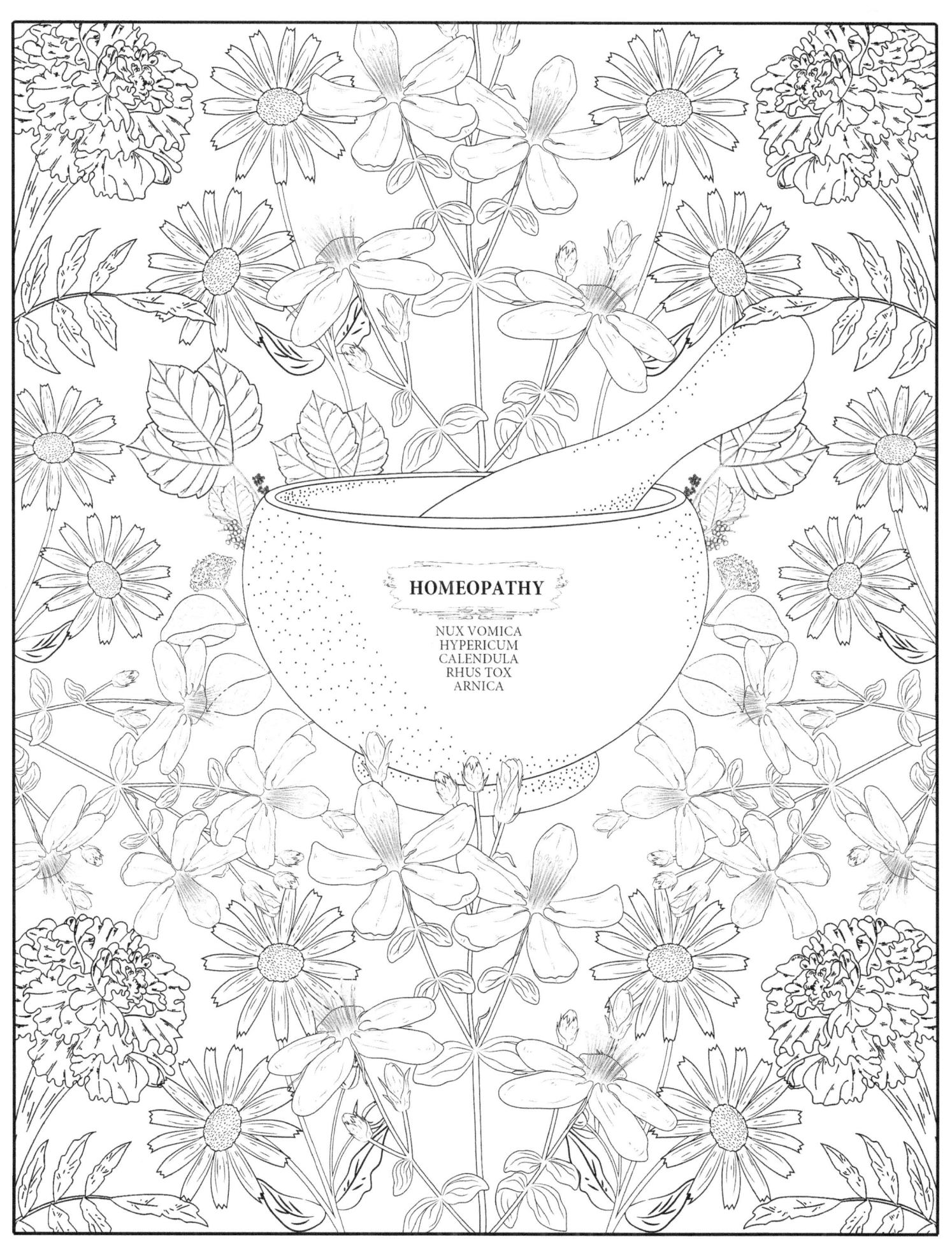

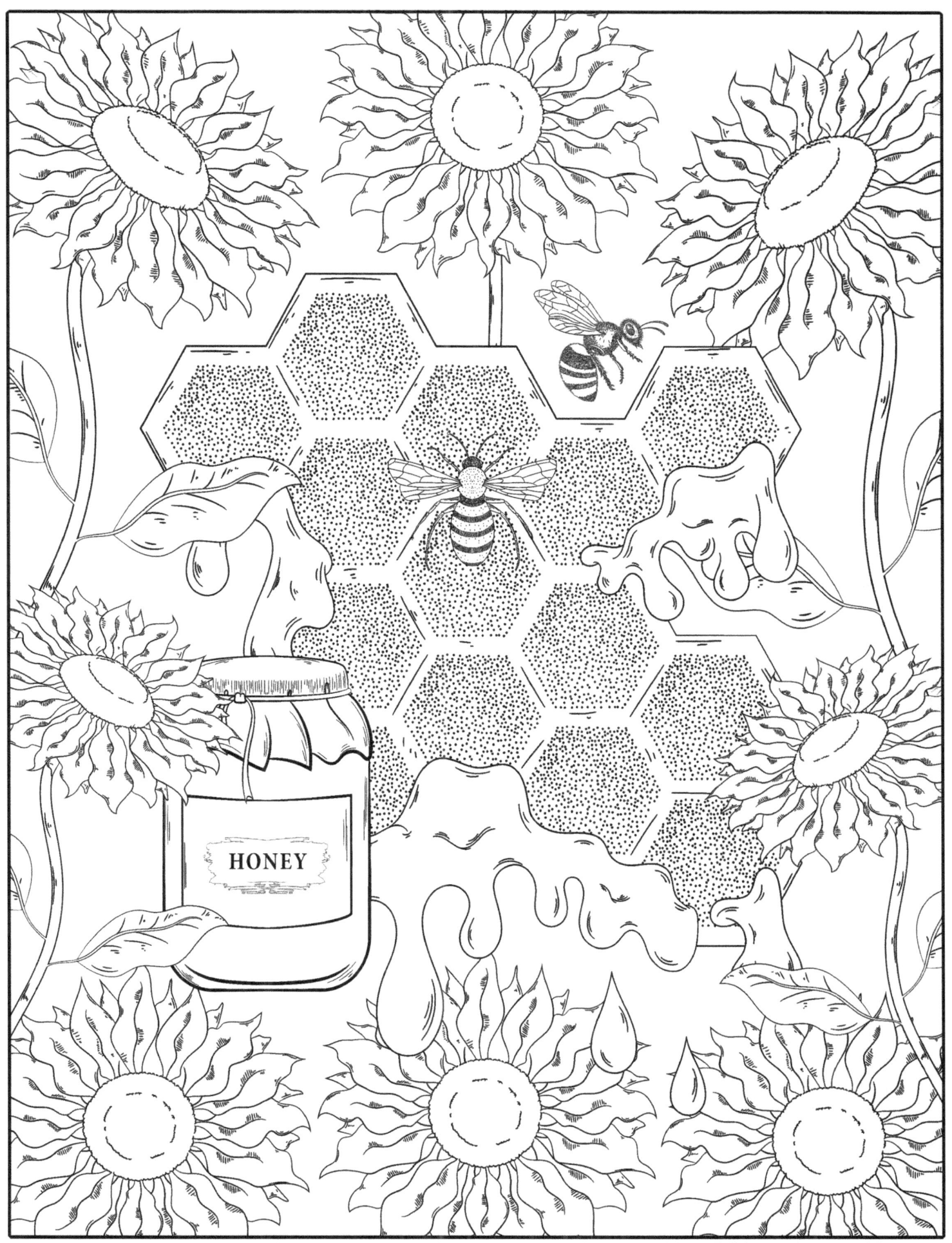

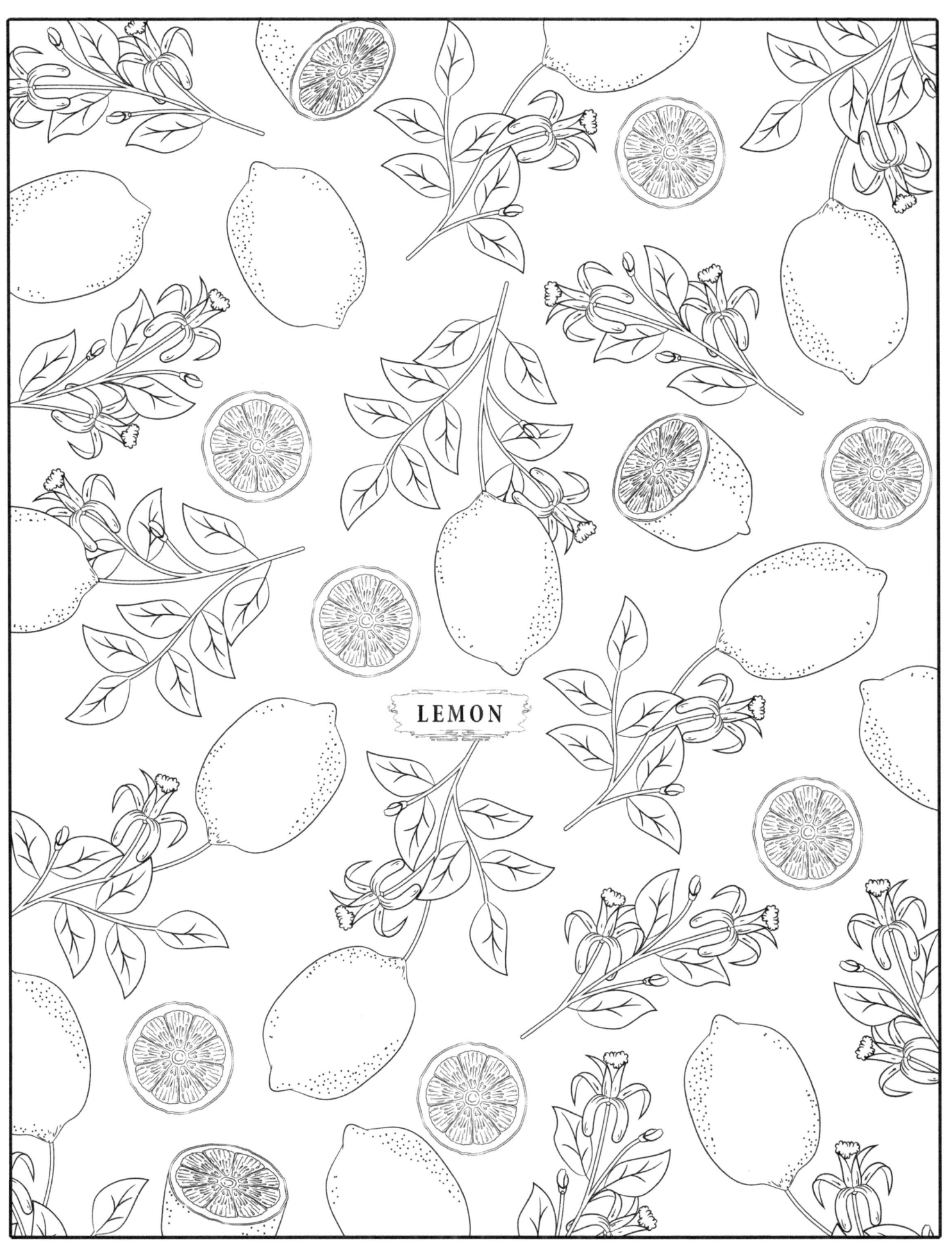

MAGNESIUM & POTASSIUM FOODS

❖ WATERMELON ❖ AVOCADOS ❖ BANANAS ❖ TOMATOES ❖ SPINACH ❖ ALMONDS ❖ SUNFLOWER SEEDS ❖ PUMPKIN SEEDS ❖

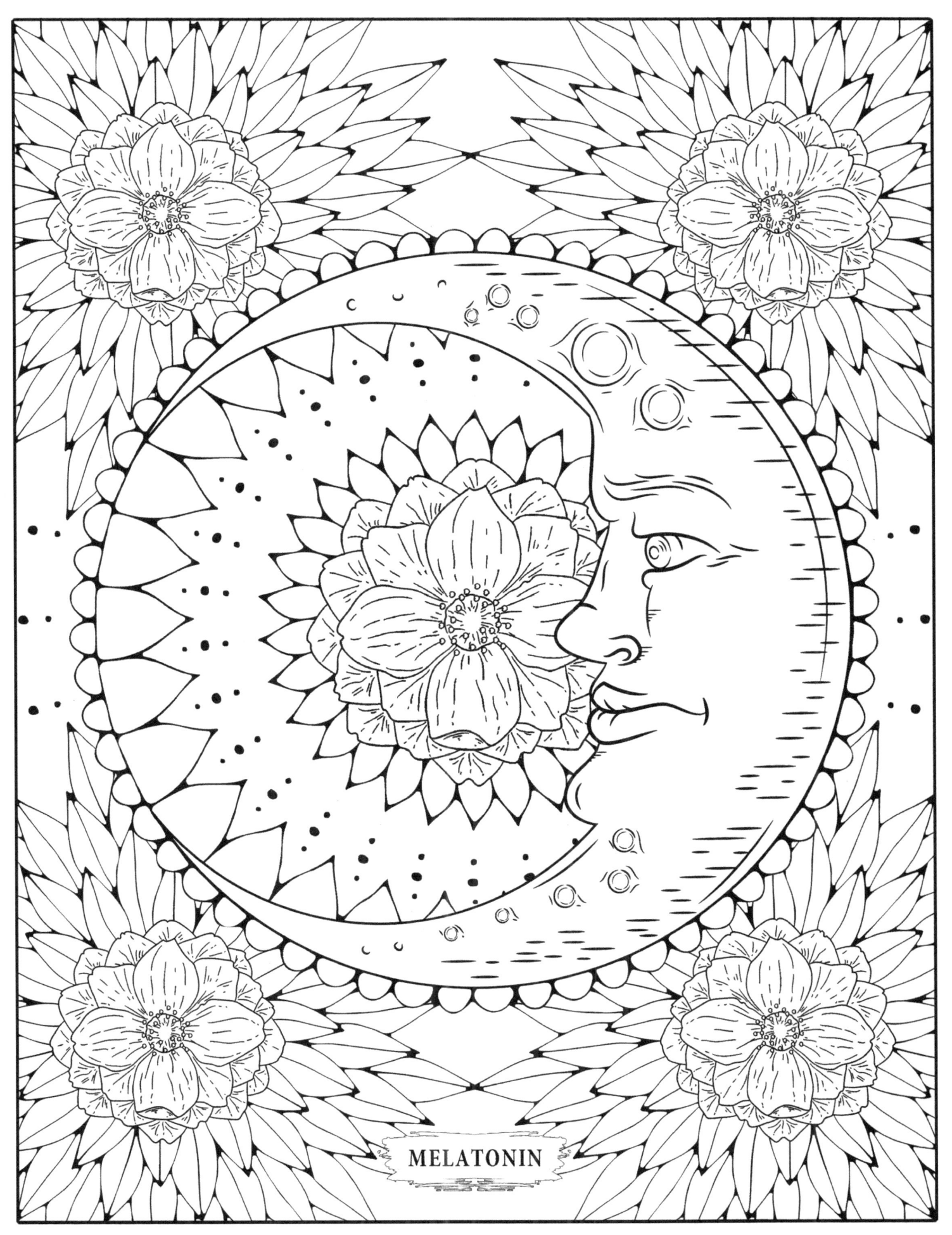

MELATONIN

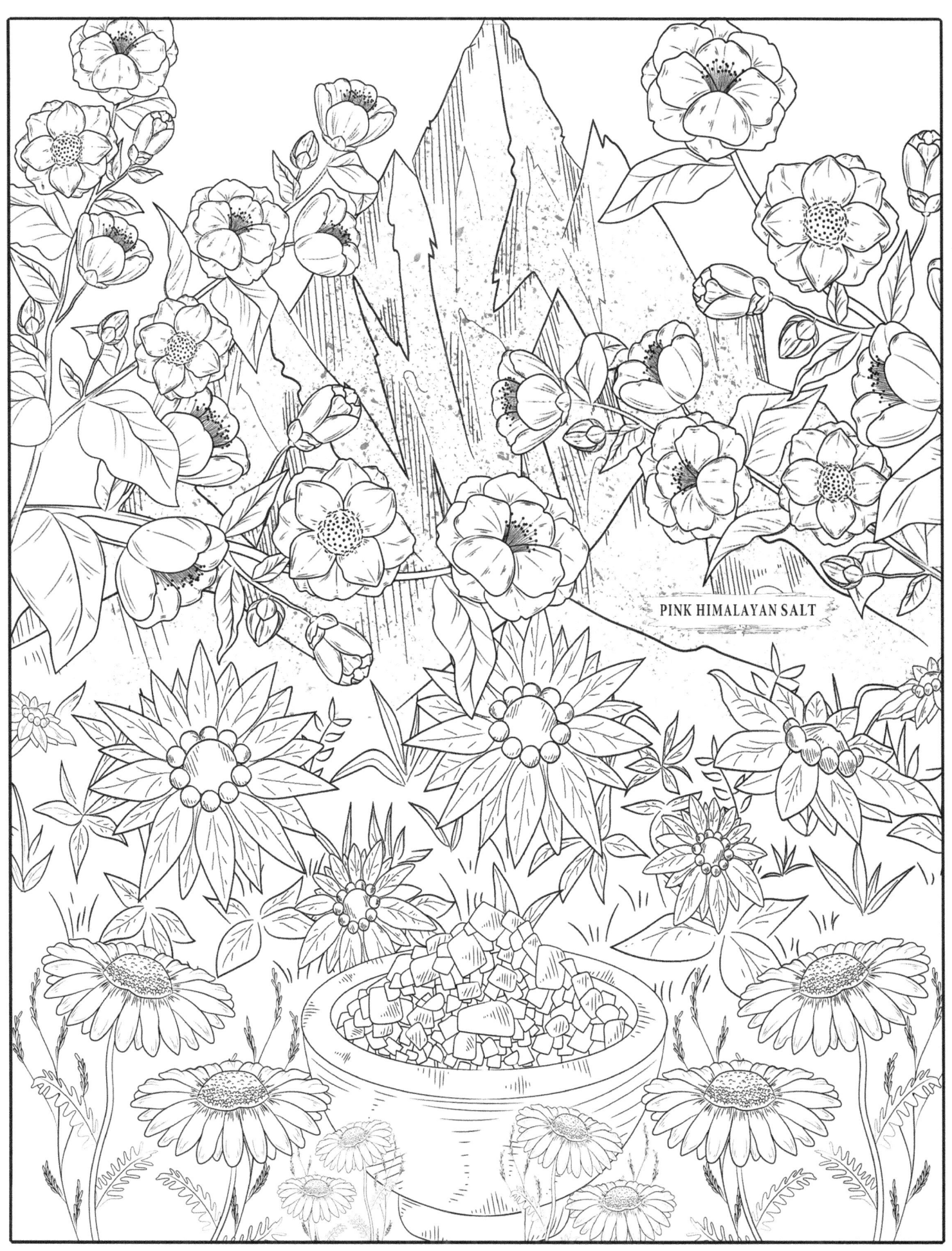

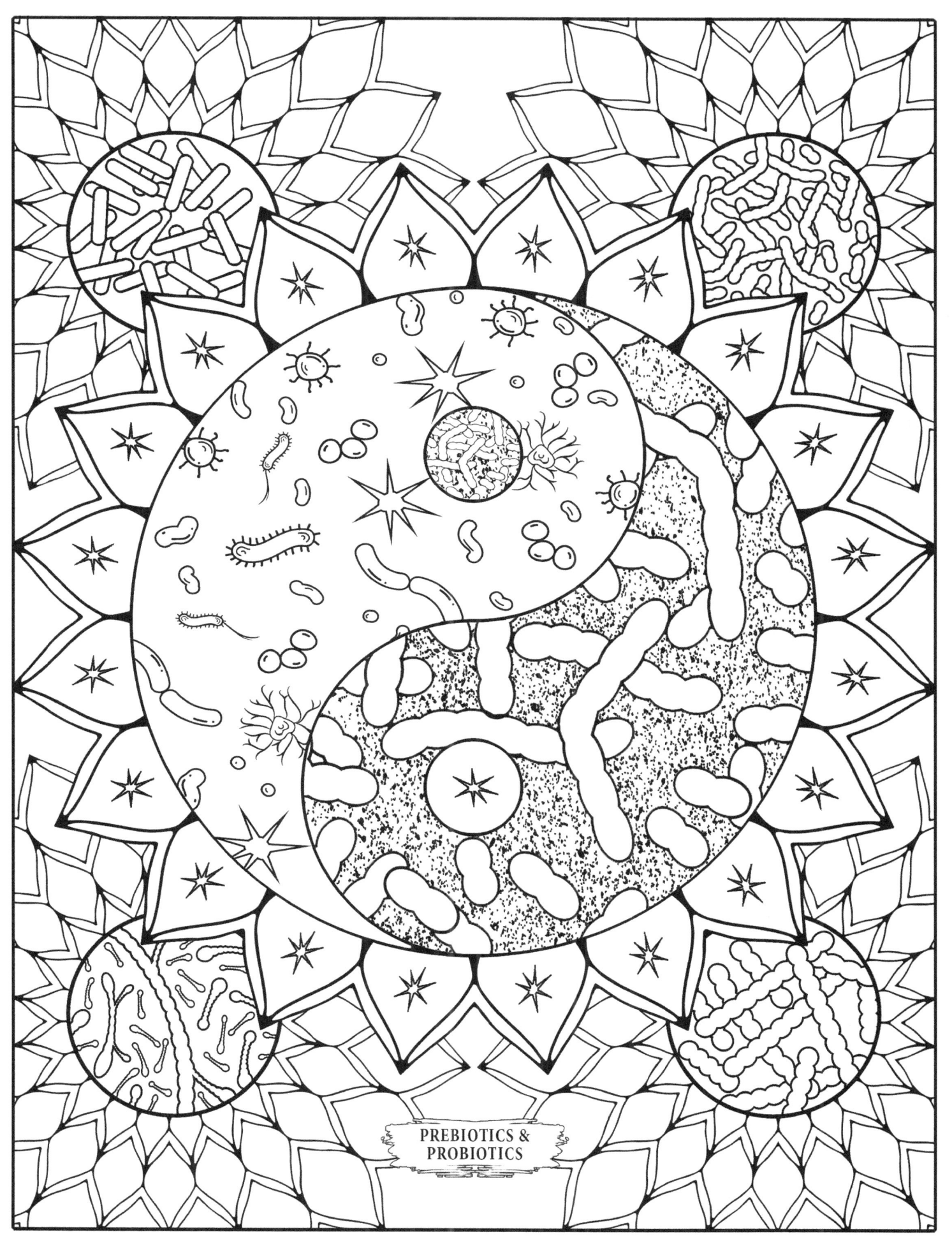

PREBIOTICS & PROBIOTICS

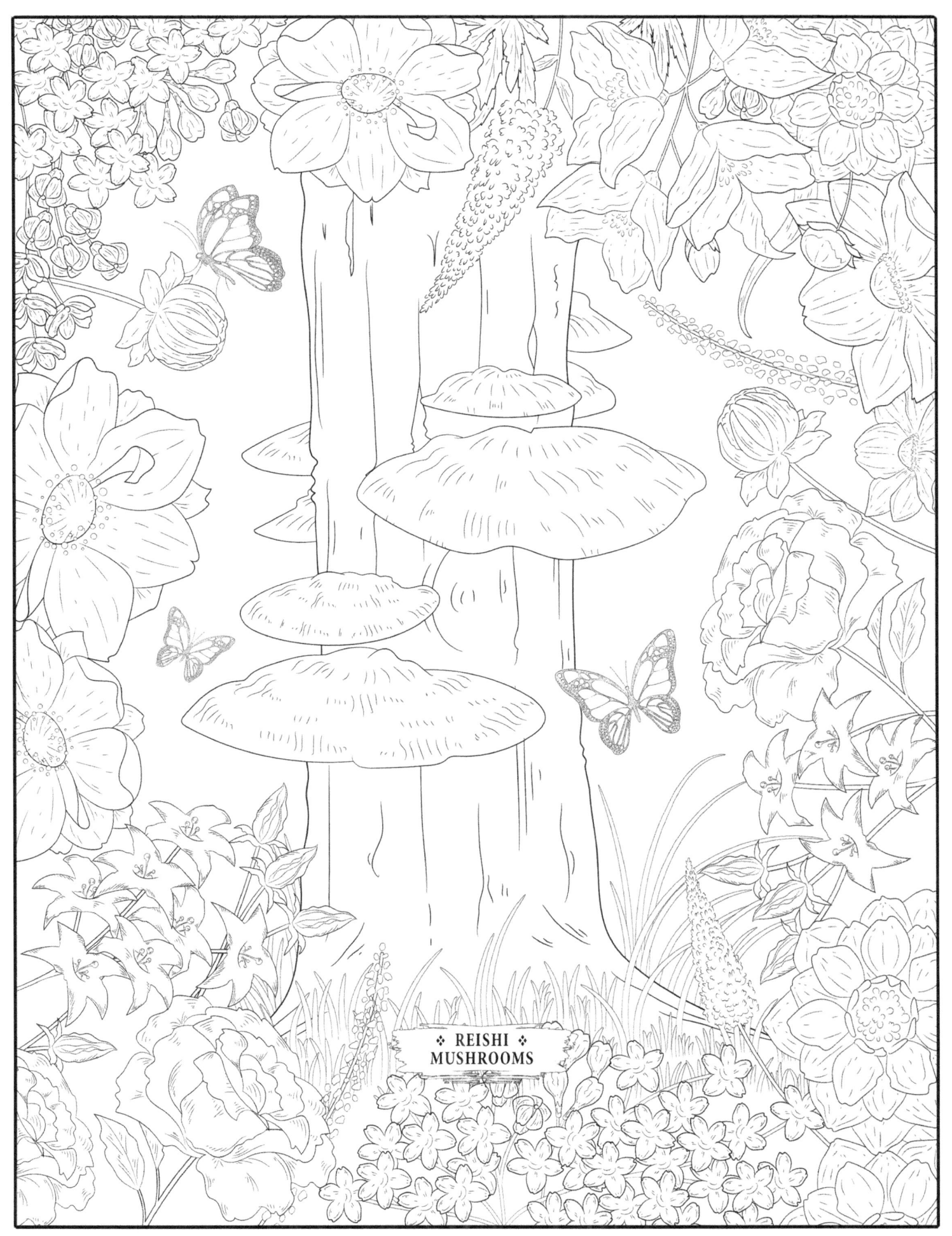

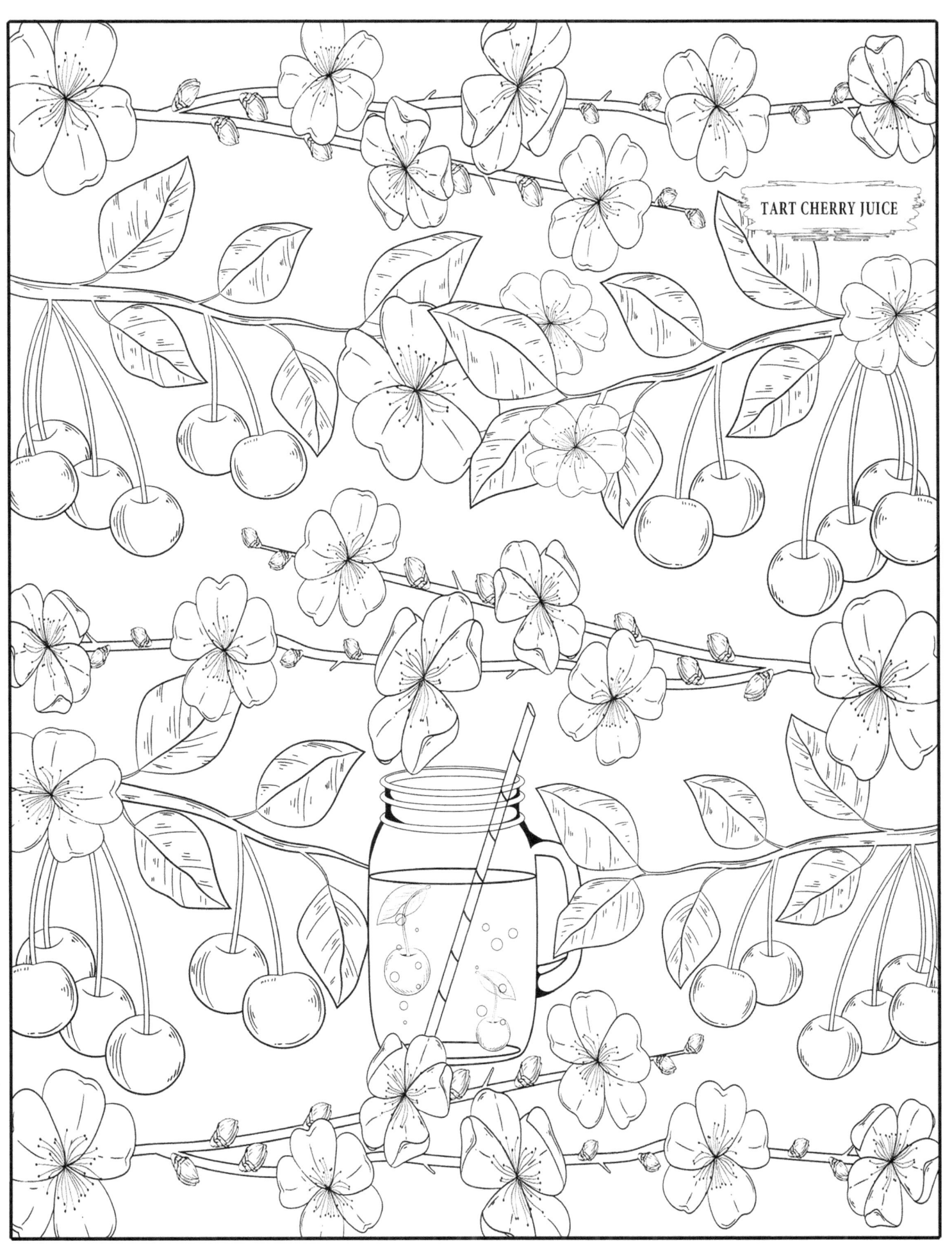

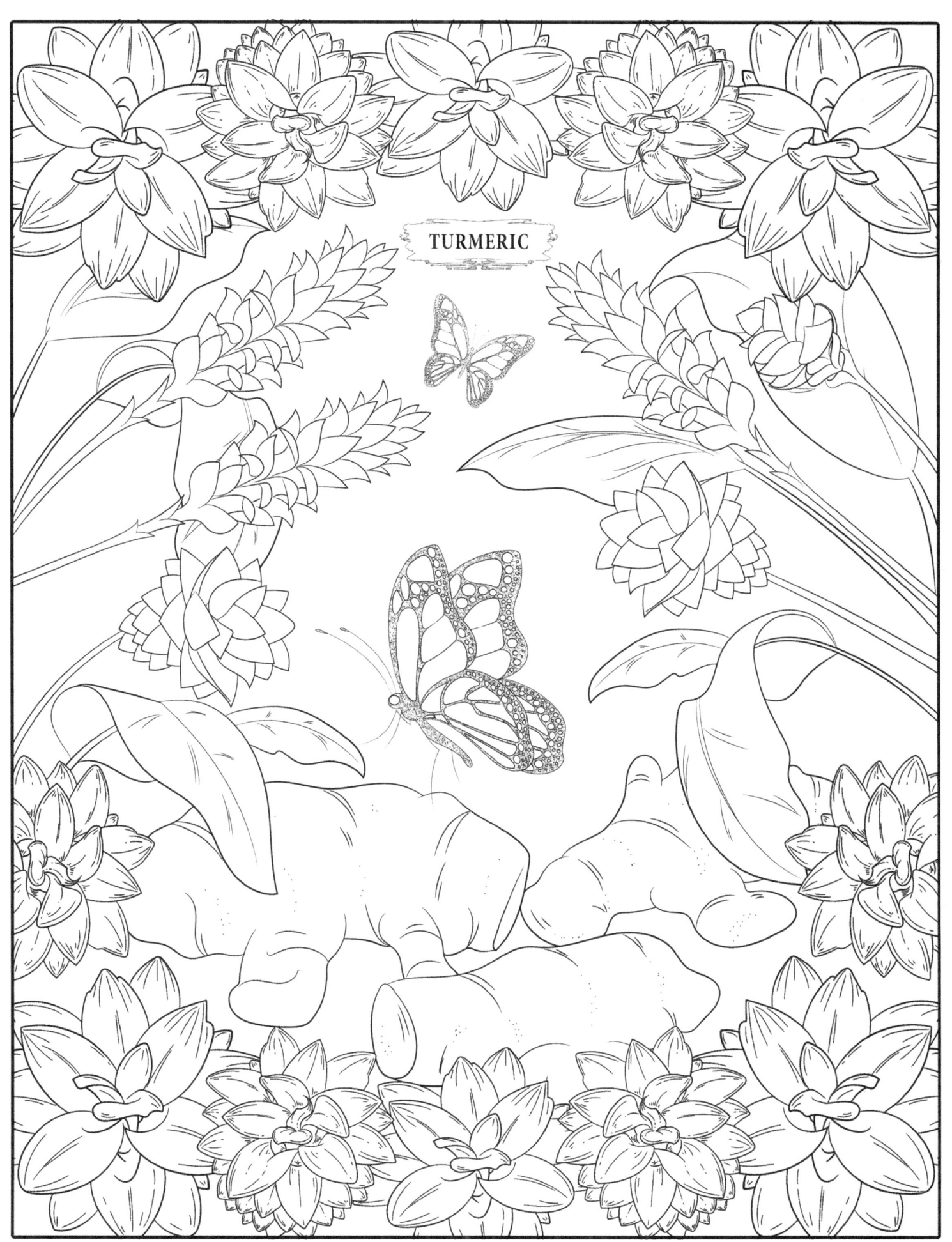

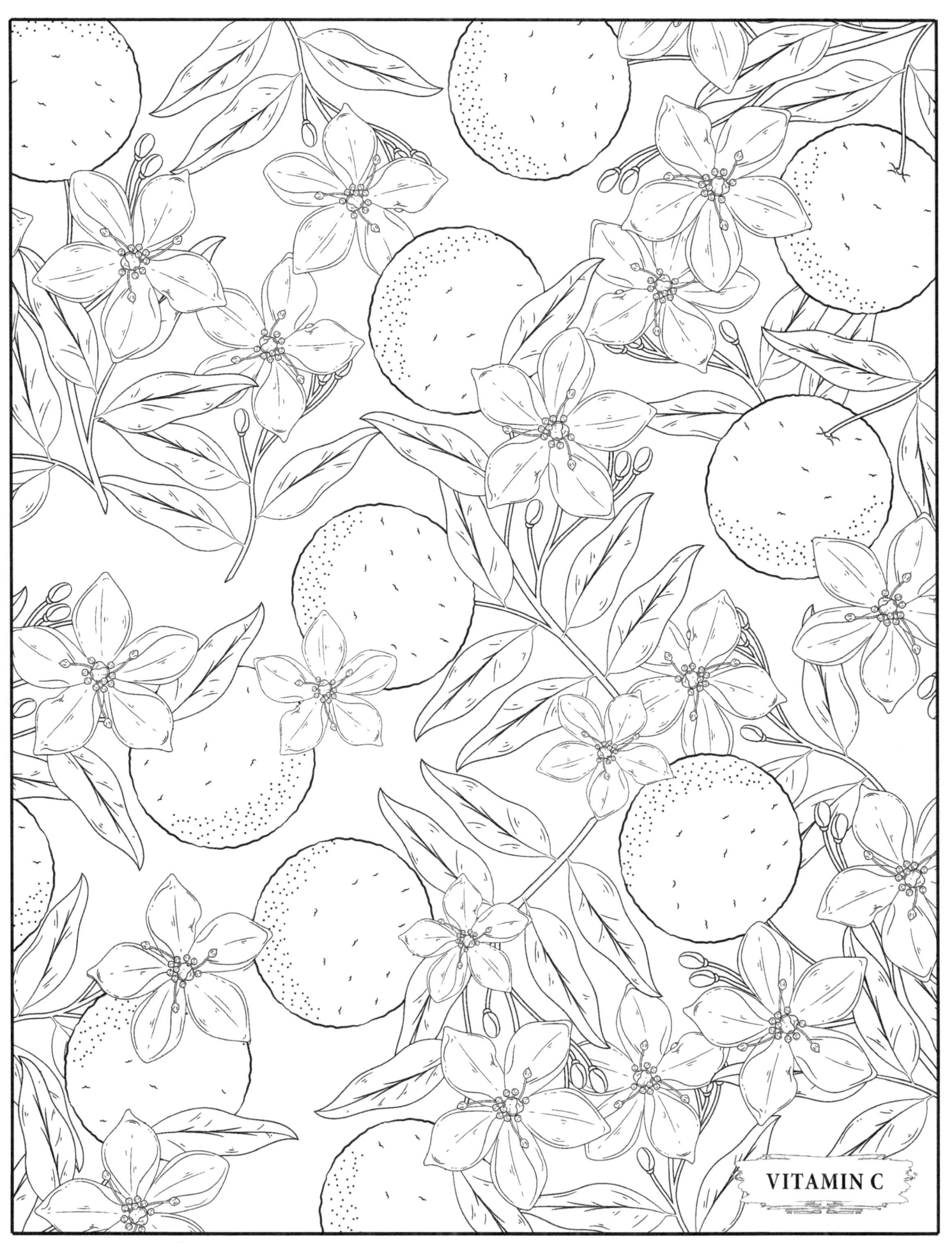